FUNGAL ARTHRITIS

Simple And Comprehensive Guide Of Treating And Overcoming Fugal Arthritis

Dr Annabel Travis

CHAPTER ONE

Introduction to Fungal Arthritis

Fungal arthritis, also known as mycotic arthritis, is a rare but serious condition characterized by inflammation of the joints resulting from fungal infection. Unlike bacterial or viral arthritis, which are more common, fungal arthritis is caused by various types of fungi infiltrating the joint space, leading to pain, swelling, and reduced mobility.

Definition of Fungal Arthritis:

Fungal arthritis occurs when fungi invade the synovial membrane, the lining of the joints, triggering an inflammatory response. This invasion can lead to the destruction of cartilage and bone within the joint, causing significant morbidity if not promptly diagnosed and treated.

Overview of Fungal Infections and Their Impact on Joints:

Fungal infections can affect various parts of the body, including the skin, lungs, and even the central nervous system. When fungi infiltrate the joints, they can cause a spectrum of symptoms ranging from mild discomfort to severe joint damage. Common fungal pathogens responsible for fungal arthritis include Candida species, Aspergillus species, and Histoplasma capsulatum.

Historical Background and Emergence of Fungal Arthritis as a Medical Concern:

The recognition of fungal arthritis as a distinct clinical entity dates back to the late 19th and early 20th centuries, with sporadic case reports highlighting the challenges in diagnosis and management. However, it was not until the latter half of the 20th century that fungal arthritis gained significant attention within the medical community, coinciding with advancements in diagnostic techniques and the emergence of immunocompromised patient populations, such as those with HIV/AIDS or undergoing immunosuppressive therapy.

The increasing prevalence of fungal infections, coupled with the growing population of individuals with compromised immune systems, has contributed to the rise in cases of fungal arthritis in recent decades. Despite advances in medical science, fungal arthritis remains a diagnostic and therapeutic challenge due to its rarity and nonspecific clinical presentation.

In the subsequent chapters, we will delve deeper into the various aspects of fungal arthritis, including its pathophysiology, diagnosis, treatment modalities, and preventive strategies, with the aim of providing clinicians, researchers, and patients with a comprehensive understanding of this intriguing yet formidable condition.

Types of fungi causing arthritis:

There are several different fungal pathogens that can cause fungal arthritis, and each one has distinct traits and clinical manifestations. Common fungi implicated in fungal arthritis include:

1. Candida species: Candida albicans is the most prevalent species responsible for fungal arthritis, particularly in immunocompromised individuals.

2. Aspergillus species: Aspergillus fumigatus and Aspergillus flavus are among the species that can cause invasive joint infections.

3. Histoplasma capsulatum: This dimorphic fungus, endemic to certain regions, can lead to joint involvement in disseminated histoplasmosis.

4. Cryptococcus neoformans: This encapsulated yeast can disseminate hematogenously and cause arthritis in immunocompromised hosts.

Pathophysiology of Fungal Arthritis:

Fungal arthritis typically occurs through hematogenous dissemination, direct inoculation, or contiguous spread from adjacent infected tissues. Once fungi gain access to the joint space, they elicit an inflammatory response characterized by synovial proliferation, neutrophil infiltration, and the release of pro-inflammatory cytokines. Fungal hyphae may invade the synovial membrane, cartilage, and bone, leading to tissue destruction and joint deformity if left untreated.

Risk Factors and Predisposing Conditions:

Several factors increase the risk of developing fungal arthritis, including:

- Immunocompromised state: Individuals with weakened immune systems, such as those with HIV/AIDS, organ transplant recipients, or patients receiving immunosuppressive therapy, are at higher risk.

- Underlying medical conditions: Chronic diseases like diabetes mellitus, rheumatoid arthritis, or systemic lupus erythematosus can predispose individuals to fungal infections, including fungal arthritis.

- Invasive procedures: Trauma, surgery, or joint injections can provide entry points for fungal pathogens to colonize and infect the joints.

- Intravenous drug use: Sharing contaminated needles or equipment can introduce fungi into the bloodstream, increasing the risk of disseminated fungal infections, including fungal arthritis.

-

Modes of Transmission and Common Sources of Infection:

Fungi causing arthritis can enter the body through various routes, including:

- Hematogenous dissemination: Fungi circulating in the bloodstream can seed the joints, particularly in immunocompromised individuals or those with fungemia.

- Direct inoculation: Trauma, surgery, or injections can introduce fungi directly into the joint space, leading to localized infection.

- Contiguous spread: Infections originating from adjacent tissues, such as osteomyelitis or soft tissue infections, can extend into the joints, causing secondary arthritis.

- Environmental exposure: Inhalation of fungal spores or contact with contaminated soil, bird droppings, or decaying organic matter can result in systemic fungal infections, including fungal arthritis.

Understanding the diverse spectrum of fungal pathogens, the pathophysiology of joint involvement, and the predisposing factors for fungal arthritis is crucial for accurate diagnosis and effective management. In the subsequent chapters, we will explore the clinical presentation, diagnostic strategies, treatment options, and preventive measures for this challenging condition.

CHAPTER TWO

Clinical Presentation and Diagnosis

Signs and Symptoms of Fungal Arthritis:

Fungal arthritis presents with a spectrum of clinical manifestations, which can vary depending on the causative organism, the duration of infection, and the host's immune status. Common signs and symptoms include:

- Joint pain: is typically localized to the affected joint(s) and may worsen with movement.

- Joint swelling: is due to inflammation and accumulation of synovial fluid.

- Limited range of motion: difficulty in moving the affected joint(s) due to pain and swelling.

- Warmth and erythema: The affected joint(s) may feel warm to the touch and appear red or inflamed.

- Systemic symptoms: fever, chills, malaise, and weight loss may accompany disseminated fungal infections.

Differential Diagnosis and Distinguishing Fungal Arthritis from Other Arthritic Conditions:

Distinguishing fungal arthritis from other causes of joint inflammation can be challenging due to overlapping clinical features. Conditions to consider in the differential diagnosis include:

- Bacterial arthritis: acute onset, severe joint pain, and systemic symptoms are more typical in bacterial arthritis.

- Viral arthritis: often presents with a prodrome of viral symptoms and may involve multiple joints.

- Rheumatoid arthritis: Chronic symmetric polyarthritis with morning stiffness is characteristic of rheumatoid arthritis.

- Crystal-induced arthritis: Gout or pseudogout can cause acute monoarthritis with characteristic joint swelling and tenderness.

Diagnostic Approaches: Laboratory Tests, Imaging Studies, and Synovial Fluid Analysis:

1. Laboratory tests:

- o Blood cultures: to detect fungemia or systemic fungal infections.

- o Fungal serology: detection of fungal antibodies or antigens in serum.

- o Complete blood count (CBC) and inflammatory markers: elevated white blood cell count and inflammatory markers (e.g., ESR, CRP) are nonspecific but may indicate ongoing infection.

2. Imaging studies:

- o X-rays: to assess for joint space narrowing, erosions, or bony destruction.

- o Magnetic resonance imaging (MRI): provides detailed visualization of soft tissue involvement and bone marrow changes.

3. Synovial fluid analysis:

- o Joint aspiration: Synovial fluid analysis for cell count, differential, Gram stain, and cultures is essential for confirming the diagnosis.

- o Fungal culture: definitive identification of the causative organism through culture of synovial fluid or tissue samples.

Challenges in Diagnosis and Potential Pitfalls:

- Non-specific presentation: Fungal arthritis can mimic other inflammatory arthropathies, delaying diagnosis and treatment.

- Low diagnostic yield of synovial fluid cultures: Fungi may be slow-growing or require specialized culture media, leading to false-negative results.

- Atypical manifestations: Fungal arthritis may present with unusual features, such as chronic indolent course or involvement of unusual joints, complicating diagnosis.

- Immunocompromised hosts: Immunocompromised patients may have atypical presentations or multiple concurrent infections, making diagnosis more challenging.

Navigating the diagnostic challenges of fungal arthritis requires a high index of suspicion, comprehensive clinical evaluation, and judicious use of diagnostic tests. Early recognition and prompt initiation of treatment are crucial to preventing joint damage and improving patient outcomes.

Epidemiology and Global Burden Prevalence of Fungal Arthritis Worldwide:

Fungal arthritis is considered a rare condition compared to other forms of arthritis, such as rheumatoid arthritis or osteoarthritis. However, its exact prevalence is challenging to determine due to underdiagnosis, particularly in regions with limited access to healthcare and diagnostic resources. Fungal arthritis accounts for a small proportion of all arthritis cases but can have significant morbidity and mortality, especially in immunocompromised individuals.

Geographic Distribution and Regional Variations:

The prevalence of fungal arthritis varies geographically, often reflecting the distribution of specific fungal pathogens and underlying risk factors. Regions with a high burden of fungal infections, such as certain parts of Africa, Asia, and Latin America, may experience a higher incidence of fungal arthritis. Endemic mycoses, such as histoplasmosis in the Ohio and Mississippi River valleys of the United States, can lead to localized clusters of fungal arthritis cases.

Impact on Different Age Groups and Demographics:

Fungal arthritis can affect individuals of all ages, but certain demographic groups may be disproportionately affected:

- Immunocompromised individuals: Patients with HIV/AIDS, organ transplant recipients, cancer patients undergoing chemotherapy, and those receiving immunosuppressive therapy are at higher risk due to impaired immune function.

- Elderly population: Age-related decline in immune function and comorbidities may predispose older adults to fungal infections, including fungal arthritis.

- Pediatric population: Although rare, fungal arthritis can occur in children, particularly in neonates with congenital immunodeficiencies or premature infants with invasive fungal infections.

Certain occupational or environmental exposures may also increase the risk of fungal arthritis. For instance, agricultural laborers exposed to contaminated soil may be more susceptible to fungal infections, such as fungal arthritis brought on by species of Coccidioides or Blastomyces dermatitidis, which are soil-dwelling fungi.

Overall, understanding the epidemiology and demographic patterns of fungal arthritis is essential for targeted surveillance, prevention efforts, and resource allocation to mitigate its impact on public health. Further research is needed to elucidate the global burden of fungal arthritis and develop strategies for early detection and management in diverse populations.

CHAPTER THREE

Treatment Strategies

Antifungal Therapy: Medications, Dosages, and Administration Routes:

Antifungal therapy is the cornerstone of treatment for fungal arthritis and aims to eradicate the causative organism while minimizing joint damage and systemic complications. Commonly used antifungal agents include:

- Azoles: Fluconazole, itraconazole, and voriconazole

- Echinocandins: Caspofungin, micafungin, and anidulafungin

Amphotericin B formulations: Lipid formulations (e.g., liposomal amphotericin B) or conventional amphotericin B

- The choice of antifungal agent depends on factors such as the identified pathogen, antifungal susceptibility, site of infection, and patient factors (e.g., renal function, drug interactions). Dosages and administration routes vary depending on the severity of infection, renal function, and formulation availability. In severe cases or those refractory to oral therapy, intravenous antifungal agents may be indicated.

-

Surgical Intervention: Indications, Procedures, and Outcomes:

Surgical intervention may be necessary in certain cases of fungal arthritis to drain abscesses, debride infected tissues, or stabilize joints. Indications for surgery include:

- Inadequate response to medical therapy

- Severe joint destruction

- Presence of abscesses or septic arthritis

Structural joint damage requiring reconstruction or arthroplasty

- Surgical procedures may include arthroscopic lavage and debridement, open surgical drainage, synovectomy, joint fusion, or joint replacement. The outcomes of surgical intervention depend on the extent of joint involvement, the timing of surgery, and the patient's overall health status.

Management of Complications and Long-Term Sequelae:

Fungal arthritis can lead to various complications and long-term sequelae, including joint deformity, chronic pain, osteomyelitis, and functional impairment. Management strategies may include:

- Physical therapy and rehabilitation: To improve joint mobility, muscle strength, and functional outcomes.

- Pain management: Analgesics, anti-inflammatory medications, or intra-articular injections may be used to alleviate pain.

- Long-term surveillance: Regular follow-up and monitoring for disease recurrence, joint damage, or complications are essential to optimize outcomes and prevent relapse.

-

Novel Approaches and Emerging Therapies:

Research into novel approaches and emerging therapies for fungal arthritis is ongoing, with several promising strategies under investigation:

- Immunomodulatory agents: Modulation of the host immune response to enhance antifungal activity and reduce inflammation.

- Targeted antifungal therapies: Development of new antifungal agents with improved efficacy, safety, and pharmacokinetic profiles.

- Adjunctive therapies: Complementary treatments such as biofilm disruptors, antifungal peptides, or immunotherapies to augment antifungal therapy and improve outcomes.

Clinical trials and translational research are needed to evaluate the safety and efficacy of these novel approaches in the management of fungal arthritis and ultimately improve patient outcomes. Close collaboration between clinicians, researchers, and industry partners is essential to advance the field of fungal arthritis treatment and address the unmet medical needs of affected individuals.

Prevention and Control

Strategies for Preventing Fungal Arthritis in High-Risk Populations:

Preventing fungal arthritis primarily involves minimizing exposure to fungal pathogens and optimizing immune function, particularly in high-risk populations. Key prevention strategies include:

- Immunization: Vaccination against specific fungal pathogens, where available, can reduce the risk of infection. For example, the histoplasmosis vaccine may be recommended for individuals at high risk of exposure in endemic areas.

- Infection control measures: Avoiding known sources of fungal exposure, such as contaminated soil or bird droppings, can help prevent fungal infections. Occupational and environmental safety protocols should be followed, especially in high-risk settings such as construction sites, farms, or healthcare facilities.

- Prophylactic antifungal therapy: To prevent invasive fungal infections, including fungal arthritis, prophylactic antifungal therapy may be indicated in certain immunocompromised populations, such as patients undergoing solid organ transplantation or hematopoietic stem cell transplantation.

- Education and awareness: Providing education and information to high-risk individuals and healthcare providers about the risks of fungal infections, preventive measures, and early signs of infection can help improve awareness and promote early intervention.

Infection Control Measures in Healthcare Settings:

In healthcare settings, preventing the nosocomial transmission of fungal pathogens is essential to protecting vulnerable patient populations. Infection control measures may include:

- Hand hygiene: Healthcare workers should adhere to strict hand hygiene protocols, including handwashing with soap and water or using alcohol-based hand sanitizers before and after patient contact.

- Environmental cleaning: Regular cleaning and disinfection of patient care areas, medical equipment, and high-touch surfaces can help reduce the risk of fungal contamination.

- Personal protective equipment (PPE): Healthcare workers should use appropriate PPE, such as gloves, gowns, masks, and eye protection, when caring for patients with suspected or confirmed fungal infections.

- Isolation precautions: Patients with known or suspected fungal infections should be placed on appropriate isolation precautions to prevent transmission to other patients and healthcare workers.

- Antifungal stewardship: Careful selection, dosing, and treatment duration in combination with antifungal agents can help prevent drug-resistant fungi from emerging and lower the risk of fungal infections linked to healthcare.

Public Health Interventions and Surveillance Programs:

Public health agencies play a crucial role in monitoring the epidemiology of fungal infections, implementing preventive measures, and responding to outbreaks. Key public health interventions may include:

- Surveillance and reporting: Establishing surveillance systems to monitor the incidence, prevalence, and trends of fungal infections, including fungal arthritis, can help identify emerging threats and inform targeted interventions.

- Outbreak investigation: Rapid response to suspected outbreaks of fungal infections in healthcare or community settings, including case identification, contact tracing, and environmental assessment, can help contain the spread of infection.

- Education and outreach: Public health campaigns aimed at raising awareness about fungal infections, risk factors, and preventive measures can empower individuals and communities to take proactive steps to protect themselves from infection.

By implementing comprehensive prevention and control strategies at the individual, healthcare, and public health levels, we can reduce the burden of fungal arthritis and improve patient outcomes. Collaboration between healthcare providers, public health agencies, policymakers, and the community is essential to effectively address the challenges posed by fungal infections and safeguard public health.

CHAPTER FOUR

Case Studies and Clinical Pearls

Real-life Cases Illustrating Diagnostic Challenges and Treatment Dilemmas:

Case Study 1:

Patient Profile: A 65-year-old male with a history of diabetes presents with progressively worsening knee pain and swelling.

Clinical Presentation: The patient reports chronic knee pain, initially attributed to osteoarthritis. However, recent worsening of symptoms and failure to respond to conventional treatments raise concerns for an alternative diagnosis.

Diagnostic Challenges: Initial evaluation reveals nonspecific inflammatory markers and inconclusive imaging findings. When a bacterial infection is ruled out by synovial fluid analysis, unusual etiologies such as fungal arthritis should be taken into account.

Treatment Dilemma: Given the possibility of drug toxicity and the absence of conclusive evidence for fungal infection, initiating empiric antifungal therapy while awaiting culture results presents difficulties. Balancing the risks and benefits of early antifungal treatment versus delayed diagnosis is crucial to optimizing patient outcomes.

Case Study 2:

Patient Profile: A 30-year-old female with rheumatoid arthritis on immunosuppressive therapy presents with acute-onset hip pain and fever.

Clinical Presentation: The patient's symptoms are initially attributed to a flare of rheumatoid arthritis. However, the rapid progression of joint symptoms and the development of systemic symptoms raise concern for septic arthritis.

Diagnostic Challenges: Blood cultures and synovial fluid analysis are negative for bacterial pathogens, prompting consideration of fungal arthritis as an alternative diagnosis. Obtaining definitive fungal cultures may be challenging due to slow growth or false-negative results.

Treatment Dilemma: Balancing the need for empiric antifungal therapy with the potential risks of prolonged immunosuppression poses a therapeutic dilemma. Close monitoring for treatment response and infectious complications is essential in guiding management decisions.

Lessons Learned and Best Practices in Managing Fungal Arthritis:

- Maintain a high index of suspicion for fungal arthritis, especially in immunocompromised patients or those with atypical clinical presentations.

- Promptly obtain synovial fluid analysis for culture and sensitivity testing in suspected cases of fungal arthritis, as early diagnosis and treatment are crucial for improving outcomes.

- Consider empiric antifungal therapy in high-risk patients with clinical suspicion of fungal arthritis, pending definitive microbiological confirmation.

- Collaborate closely with infectious disease specialists and rheumatologists to optimize diagnostic and treatment strategies for fungal arthritis in complex cases.

- Educate patients and caregivers about the importance of adherence to antifungal therapy, regular follow-up, and early recognition of signs of treatment failure or disease recurrence.

Complications and Outcomes:

- complications of fungal arthritis may include joint destruction, chronic pain, functional impairment, and systemic dissemination.

- Long-term outcomes depend on factors such as the underlying immune status, promptness of diagnosis and treatment, extent of joint involvement, and response to therapy.

- Delayed diagnosis and inadequate treatment may result in irreversible joint damage and poor functional outcomes.

- Close monitoring for complications, such as relapse of infection, development of secondary osteomyelitis, or drug-related adverse effects, is essential to optimize patient outcomes and quality of life.

By sharing real-life case studies, clinical pearls, and lessons learned, clinicians can enhance their understanding of the diagnostic and therapeutic challenges associated with fungal arthritis and improve patient care and outcomes. Ongoing research and collaboration are essential to advance our knowledge of this complex condition and develop more effective management strategies.

Future Directions and Research Perspectives

Ongoing Research Initiatives and Areas of Investigation:

1. Pathogenesis Studies: Investigating the host-pathogen interactions and immune responses involved in fungal arthritis to identify novel therapeutic targets and diagnostic biomarkers.

2. Antifungal Drug Development: Developing new antifungal agents with enhanced efficacy, safety profiles, and novel mechanisms of action to combat drug-resistant fungi and improve treatment outcomes.

3. Diagnostic Advances: Exploring novel diagnostic modalities, such as molecular assays, proteomics, and imaging techniques, to enhance the accuracy and timeliness of fungal arthritis diagnosis.

4. Host Susceptibility Factors: Understanding genetic, immunological, and environmental factors that predispose individuals to fungal arthritis informs targeted preventive strategies and personalized treatment approaches.

5. Epidemiological Surveillance: Conducting population-based studies and surveillance programs to monitor the epidemiology, trends, and geographic distribution of fungal arthritis and identify emerging threats.

Promising Avenues for Improving Diagnosis, Treatment, and Prevention:

1. Point-of-Care Diagnostics: Developing rapid, point-of-care diagnostic tests for fungal arthritis that can be readily implemented in resource-limited settings to facilitate early diagnosis and prompt initiation of treatment.

2. Immunotherapeutic Approaches: Harnessing the host immune response through immunomodulatory agents, monoclonal antibodies, or adoptive cell therapies to enhance antifungal activity and reduce inflammation in fungal arthritis.

3. Precision Medicine: Advancing precision medicine approaches to tailor antifungal therapy based on individual patient factors, including genetic predisposition, immune status, and fungal susceptibility profiles.

4. Targeted Drug Delivery: Designing targeted drug delivery systems, such as nanoparticles or liposomes, to improve the efficacy, bioavailability, and tissue penetration of antifungal agents while minimizing systemic toxicity.

5. Vaccination Strategies: Developing vaccines against specific fungal pathogens implicated in fungal arthritis to prevent infection and reduce the burden of disease in high-risk populations.

6.

Collaboration Opportunities and Interdisciplinary Approaches:

1. Translational Research: Fostering collaboration between basic scientists, clinicians, and industry partners to translate fundamental discoveries into clinical applications and novel therapeutics for fungal arthritis.

2. Multidisciplinary Care Teams: Establishing multidisciplinary care teams comprising infectious disease specialists, rheumatologists, orthopedic surgeons, microbiologists, and immunologists to optimize patient management and outcomes.

3. Global Health Partnerships: Strengthening international collaborations and partnerships to

address the global burden of fungal arthritis, particularly in resource-limited settings where access to diagnostics and treatment is limited.

4. Patient Engagement: Engaging patients, advocacy organizations, and community stakeholders in research, education, and advocacy efforts to raise awareness, improve access to care, and empower individuals affected by fungal arthritis.

5. Education and Training: Providing training and educational resources for healthcare providers, researchers, and policymakers to enhance their understanding of fungal arthritis and promote evidence-based practices in diagnosis, treatment, and prevention.

By fostering collaboration, advancing innovative research, and embracing interdisciplinary approaches, we can accelerate progress in the prevention, diagnosis, and treatment of fungal arthritis, ultimately improving patient outcomes and reducing the global burden of this challenging condition.

CHAPTER FIVE

Patient Education and Advocacy

Resources for Patients and Caregivers:

1. Patient Information Materials: Providing patients and caregivers with educational materials, brochures, and pamphlets explaining fungal arthritis, its causes, symptoms, diagnosis, and treatment options.

2. Online Resources: Curating reputable websites, forums, and online communities where patients can access reliable information, connect with others facing similar challenges, and seek support and advice.

3. Educational Workshops: organizing educational workshops or webinars led by healthcare professionals to address common questions and concerns related to fungal arthritis and empower patients to become active participants in their care.

4. Patient Navigators: Offering the support of patient navigators or care coordinators who can guide

patients through the healthcare system, provide personalized assistance, and connect them with relevant resources and services.

Support groups and advocacy organizations:

1. Patient Support Groups: Facilitating the formation of patient support groups or peer-to-peer networks where individuals affected by fungal arthritis can share experiences, exchange information, and offer mutual support and encouragement.

2. Advocacy Organizations: Partnering with advocacy organizations dedicated to raising awareness, promoting research, and advocating for policies that improve access to care, funding for research, and quality of life for patients with fungal arthritis.

3. Online Communities: Engaging with online communities and social media platforms where patients, caregivers, and advocates can connect, share resources, raise awareness, and advocate for the needs of the fungal arthritis community.

4. Public Awareness Campaigns: Collaborating with advocacy organizations to launch public awareness campaigns, events, and initiatives aimed at educating the public, policymakers, and healthcare providers about the impact of fungal

arthritis and the importance of early detection
and treatment.

Empowering Patients to Play an Active Role in Their Care:

1. Patient Education Programs: Offering educational programs and workshops that empower patients to become informed advocates for their own health, understand their treatment options, and actively participate in shared decision-making with their healthcare providers.

2. Self-Management Strategies: Providing patients with tools, resources, and strategies for self-management, including lifestyle modifications, symptom monitoring, medication adherence, and communication skills for navigating the healthcare system.

3. Shared Decision-Making: encouraging shared decision-making between patients and healthcare providers, where patients are actively involved in treatment decisions, goal setting, and care planning based on their preferences, values, and priorities.

4. Health Literacy Initiatives: Promoting health literacy initiatives that improve patients'

understanding of medical terminology, treatment regimens, and healthcare information empowers them to make informed decisions and advocate for their health needs.

By empowering patients and caregivers with knowledge, resources, and support, we can enhance their ability to navigate the challenges of fungal arthritis, access appropriate care, and actively engage in their treatment and management journey. We can improve outcomes and quality of life for individuals with fungal arthritis by raising awareness, amplifying patient voices, and enacting positive change through community partnerships and advocacy efforts.

In conclusion, fungal arthritis represents a complex and often overlooked condition that poses diagnostic, therapeutic, and public health challenges. Throughout this book, we have explored various aspects of fungal arthritis, including its epidemiology, clinical presentation, diagnosis, treatment, prevention, and patient advocacy. Here is a recap of key points discussed:

- Fungal arthritis is a rare but serious condition characterized by joint inflammation resulting from fungal infection, with Candida, Aspergillus, and

Histoplasma among the common causative agents.

- diagnosis of fungal arthritis can be challenging due to nonspecific symptoms, overlapping clinical features with other arthritic conditions, and limitations in diagnostic tests.

- Treatment involves antifungal therapy, often in combination with surgical intervention in severe cases, with a focus on early diagnosis and prompt initiation of therapy to prevent joint damage and systemic complications.

- Prevention strategies include infection control measures, immunization, and patient education, with a need for increased awareness and surveillance efforts to address the global burden of fungal arthritis.

Addressing fungal arthritis as a public health priority is crucial for improving outcomes and reducing the morbidity and mortality associated with this condition. By raising awareness, enhancing diagnostic capabilities, expanding treatment options, and promoting patient advocacy, we can advance efforts to combat fungal infections of the joints. However, challenges remain, including the need for improved diagnostics, access to care, and research into novel therapeutic approaches.

Looking ahead, opportunities abound for interdisciplinary collaboration, innovation, and advocacy to address the multifaceted challenges of fungal arthritis. By harnessing the collective expertise of healthcare providers, researchers, policymakers, advocacy organizations, and patients, we can drive progress in the prevention, diagnosis, and treatment of fungal infections of the joints, ultimately improving the lives of individuals affected by this complex and often debilitating condition.

As we continue to learn and evolve in our understanding of fungal arthritis, let us remain committed to advancing science, promoting patient-centered care, and advocating for policies and initiatives that prioritize the health and well-being of those living with fungal arthritis. Together, we can make a meaningful impact in the fight against fungal infections of the joints and pave the way for a healthier future for all.